BUILDING BROKEN BONES

HEALTHY LIFESTYLE WITHIN THE PERFECT SYSTEM

BY

DR. BEN JAPHETH

TABLE OF CONTENTS

Introduction

Effective fitness is an important tool for a healthy life. Regular exercise is proven to ameliorate physical and internal health, reduce the threat of habitual conditions, and enhance overall quality of life. Engaging in physical exertion releases feel-good hormones that boost mood and energy situations. also, it plays an essential part in maintaining healthy body weight and reducing the liability of rotundity- related conditions. also, a regular fitness authority can ameliorate sleep quality, drop stress situations, and enhance cognitive function. Making fitness a precedence is critical to promote the well- being of the mind and body. - Grounded on a study published in the British Journal of Sports Medicine, regular exercise can reduce the threat of habitual conditions, similar as heart complaint, stroke, and diabetes. - A study from Harvard Medical School set up that indeed moderate exercise can ameliorate sleep quality and reduce the symptoms of anxiety and depression. Regular physical exercise has a myriad of benefits for physical and internal health. still, certain types of fitness training can lead to common degeneration over time. This occurs when inordinate force and repetitious movement cause damage to the cartilage, ligaments, and other structures in and around the joints. High- impact exercises like running, jumping, and plyometrics can be particularly hard on joints, as can heavy toning with poor form. Without proper rest and recovery time, the body's natural form processes can not keep up with the damage being done, leading to long- term joint problems.   It's important to balance fitness training with low- impact exercise and rest days to avoid common degeneration and injury. Also, proper form, fashion, and outfit can help minimise the threat of common damage.

CHAPTER 1

POSTURE IMPROVEMENT

Posture Improvement: The Key to Healthy Living

Posture is a pivotal aspect of our everyday lives because it's a abecedarian body language signal that sends dispatches to the world about ourselves. It affects not only our physical health but also our emotional well- being and confidence. numerous people suffer from poor posture due to the dragged sitting habits and sedentary life that have come the norm in ultramodern society. Fortunately, there are several ways to ameliorate our posture that can lead to a better quality of life.   One of the most effective ways to ameliorate posture is through regular exercise. Physical exertion is essential to strengthen the muscles responsible for maintaining good posture, similar as the core muscles in the tummy and back. Conditioning like yoga, Pilates, and weight training can help develop proper alignment and balance, leading to better posture. Regular exercise can also help manage weight, reducing the threat of rotundity, and other health problems that can affect posture.   Another way to ameliorate posture is by making simple changes to our diurnal routine. For illustration, sitting up straight with the shoulders squared and the reverse straight can help align the chine rightly. When standing, the weight should be balanced unevenly between both bases, with the knees slightly fraudulent to reduce pressure on the lower reverse. Avoiding high heels and inordinate use of handheld bias has also been shown to ameliorate posture significantly. These small life changes can go a long way in enhancing our posture and overall well-being. likewise, posture can be bettered by taking regular breaks when seated or standing for dragged ages. Throughout the day, taking small breaks and stretching can help palliate pressure and muscle stiffness, which can negatively impact posture over time. Simple exercises like shoulder rolls, torso twists, and neck stretches can help muscle soreness while promoting better posture. also, proper ergonomics can contribute to posture enhancement. Poor work conditions similar as unsupportive chairpersons or indecorous office height can beget or aggravate poor posture. Setting up an ergonomic workstation with a probative president, office, and computer screen can limit muscular strain and allow for proper alignment of the chine, reducing the threat of poor posture. Corrective bias can also help support good posture habits. bias like posture braces, shirts, and belts can promote healthy spinal alignment by helping to keep the shoulders pulled back and the reverse straight. These bias are particularly useful for those who spend a lot of time sitting, driving, or doing other sedentary conditioning. While posture enhancement can have a significant impact on our physical health, it also affects our emotional well- being and tone- confidence. Proper posture can boost tone- regard, enhance mood, and reduce stress situations by perfecting breathing and rotation. When the body is rightly aligned, it works efficiently, leading to increased energy situations and productivity.   In conclusion, perfecting posture is essential for maintaining overall health and well- being. Through regular exercise, administering good habits, taking frequent breaks, icing proper ergonomics, and using corrective bias, we can ameliorate posture and help musculoskeletal diseases associated with poor posture. The capability to maintain good posture not only promotes physical health but also boosts confidence, mood, and productivity. thus, incorporating posture enhancement ways into diurnal life and taking small way to ameliorate posture can have significant long- term benefits.

CHAPTER 2

EXERCISE TO STOP PAIN IN JOINT

Exercise to Stop Pains in Joints

Common pain is a common condition that affects people of all periods. It can be caused by colourful factors, including injury, arthritis, and overuse. common pain can limit your mobility and affect your quality of life, but regular exercise can help manage the pain and ameliorate your common health. In this essay, I'll bandy the benefits of exercise for common pain and give some examples of exercises to stop pains in joints. Exercising regularly has been shown to have a positive impact on common health. In fact, a study conducted by the Arthritis Foundation stated that exercise can help reduce joint pain and stiffness while also perfecting inflexibility, strength, and balance. The study also set up that exercise can help ameliorate mood and reduce the threat of depression in people with common pain. One of the stylish types of exercise for common pain is low-impact exercise. Low- impact exercises are gentle on the joints, making them a great option for people with common pain. Walking, swimming, and biking are each great exemplifications of low- impact exercises that can help ameliorate common health. Walking is one of the easiest and most accessible forms of exercise, and it can be done anywhere at any time. Walking helps ameliorate common inflexibility, reduce stiffness, and increase blood inflow to the joints. It's important to start sluggishly and traditionally make up to longer walks to avoid overstating it and causing further pain. Walking on a flat face is also recommended to reduce the impact on the joints.   Swimming is another great low-impact exercise that can help relieve common pain. The buoyancy of the water helps support the body and reduces the impact on the joints. Swimming can also help ameliorate muscle strength and inflexibility, which can further reduce common pain.However, consider taking a class or working with a syncope trainer to learn proper form and fashion, If you're new to swimming. Biking is another excellent low- impact exercise that can help reduce joint pain. Biking helps ameliorate common mobility, reduce stiffness, and increase overall fitness. It's important to acclimate the bike to your specific requirements and capacities to help prevent pain and injury.   Strength training is another important element of exercise for common pain. Structure muscle strength helps support the joints and ameliorate overall function. Resistance bands, free weights, and weight machines are   each great options for strength training. It's important to start with light weights and gradually work up to heavier weights to avoid injury.   Stretching is also salutary for common pain. Stretching helps ameliorate common inflexibility, reduce stiffness, and ameliorate overall mobility. Yoga and Pilates are both excellent options for incorporating stretching into your exercise routine.   When starting an exercise program, it's important to start sluggishly and traditionally make up for further violent exercises. It's also important to hear to your body and stop if you witness pain during exercise.However, it's important to see a croaker or physical therapist to determine the underpinning cause of the pain and admit applicable treatment, If you witness patient common pain. In conclusion, exercise can be an effective way to manage common pain and ameliorate overall   common health. Low- impact exercises similar to walking, swimming, and biking, as well as strength training and stretching, can all help reduce joint pain and stiffness. It's important to start sluggishly and traditionally make up to further violent exercises to avoidinjury.However, it's important to see a croaker or physical therapist for applicable treatment, If you witness patient common pain.

CHAPTER 3

HOW TO BUILD YOUR MUSCLES

Ways to Build Muscles: An Overview

Building muscle takes time, dedication, and, above all, consistency. It is essential to understand the basics of muscle building, including nutrition, exercise, and rest, in order to achieve your goals. In this essay, we will explore the various ways to build muscles.

First and foremost, nutrition plays a vital role in building muscles. Maintaining a balanced diet, providing enough protein, and proper hydration are all crucial factors. Protein is required for muscle growth, and it is necessary to consume enough protein to meet your needs. According to the International Society of Sports Nutrition, it is recommended to consume 1.4-2.0 grams of protein per kilogram of body weight for muscle growth in adults(1). In addition, a sufficient intake of carbohydrates and fats is necessary to provide the energy for workouts and for growth.

Secondly, regular exercise that involves weights and resistance training is crucial for building muscles. Resistance training such as free weights, machines, or bodyweight exercises, help put stress on muscles and cause them to grow. Additionally, doing compound movements such as squats, deadlifts, bench press, and pull-ups that involve more than one muscle group are effective at building muscle mass. It is essential to start with low weight and gradually increase the weights as you get stronger. Over time, progressive overload is the key to building muscle effectively.

Thirdly, rest and recovery are equally important aspects of muscle building as exercise and nutrition. Sleep and rest are essential, as the muscles require time to repair and grow. Adequate rest between workouts is necessary to allow the muscles to recover from the previous workout. Overtraining may lead to muscle breakdown instead of building and therefore hinder progress. Therefore, it is crucial to allow enough time between training sessions for muscle recovery.

Fourthly, supplements may aid in building muscle mass, however they should be viewed with caution. Some supplements claim to help build muscle but may not be effective or safe. However, there are supplements such as creatine, protein powders, and branched-chain amino acids (BCAAs), that have been studied for their effectiveness in aiding muscle growth. According to the National Academy of Sports Medicine, protein powders and BCAAs can be beneficial, especially for those who may struggle to consume enough protein in their diets(2). It is important to note that supplements should be used with care and should not replace a healthy diet.

In conclusion, there are several ways to build muscles, including nutrition, exercise, recovery, and supplementation. It is essential to remain consistent and dedicated to the process and to progress gradually over time. Building muscle takes time and effort but with a balanced approach, it is within reach.

CHAPTER 4

WAYS TO INCREASE STRENGTH

Strength is a crucial aspect of physical fitness since it not only improves one's health but also enables one to perform tasks more effectively. While some individuals may become stronger naturally due to genetic factors, most people must work hard to increase their strength. This article will highlight some of the effective ways to increase strength.

Firstly, lifting weights is one of the best ways to increase strength. Resistance training, also known as weight lifting or strength training, involves the use of weights to increase muscle mass and strength. Studies have shown that weight lifting, even with light weights, can lead to significant strength gains in both men and women. However, to achieve optimal results, one needs to lift heavier weights progressively, which helps to stimulate muscle growth. It is also essential to have a good form while lifting weights to prevent injuries and ensure that the right muscles are targeted.

Secondly, incorporating compound exercises into your workout routine can also help to increase strength. Compound exercises are those that work multiple muscle groups simultaneously, such as squats, deadlifts, and bench presses. These exercises not only enhance muscular strength but also improve overall physical fitness. By performing compound exercises, one can increase muscle mass, improve flexibility, and enhance cardiovascular health. It is also essential to progressively add weights to these exercises to provide resistance and stimulate muscle growth.

Thirdly, consuming a sufficient amount of protein is critical for muscle growth and strength development. Protein is a nutrient that serves as the building block for muscles. Therefore, consuming enough protein can help maintain and increase muscle mass, which can translate into increased strength. Studies have shown that individuals who consume high-protein diets experience more significant muscle growth when engaging in strength training. Experts recommend that one should consume 1.6 grams of protein per kilogram of body weight per day to promote muscle growth and strength development.

Fourthly, getting enough rest and sleep is essential for strength development. During exercise, the muscles undergo wear and tear, which results in muscle fatigue. Resting helps to give the muscles sufficient time to recover and repair themselves, which stimulates muscle growth and development. It is also vital to get enough sleep since this is the time when the muscles undergo repair and growth. Experts recommend that one should get at least seven hours of sleep per night to promote muscle growth and overall health.

Fifthly, taking supplements such as creatine and beta-alanine can enhance strength development. Creatine is a natural compound that is present in the body and is responsible for supplying energy to the muscles. By taking creatine supplements, one can increase the amount of creatine in the muscles, which can result in more prolonged and intense workouts. Beta-alanine, on the other hand, is an amino acid that is responsible for reducing muscle fatigue. By taking beta-alanine supplements, one can delay the onset of muscle fatigue, enabling them to perform more reps and sets, which can translate to increased strength.

Lastly, tracking progress is crucial for strength development. By monitoring progress, one can determine whether they are making progress or not and adjust their workout routine accordingly. It is essential to keep track of the weight that one is lifting, the number of reps performed, and how frequently one is performing different exercises. By doing this, one can make informed decisions regarding their training routine and make the necessary changes to achieve maximum strength development.

In conclusion, there are several effective ways to increase strength. Lifting weights, incorporating compound exercises, consuming enough protein, resting sufficiently, taking supplements, and tracking progress are some of the best ways to increase strength. However, it is essential to note that these methods require consistency and dedication to achieve optimal results. By following these guidelines, one can achieve significant strength gains and improve their overall health and fitness.

CHAPTER 5

FORTIFY YOUR JOINT AT ANY AGE

Joints are the point of contact between two or more bones in the human body. They are responsible for facilitating a range of movements, such as walking, running, jumping, and bending. However, as we age, our joints undergo wear and tear, resulting in joint pain and stiffness. Fortifying your joint is essential because it reduces the risk of joint injury, slows down the degenerative process, and improves overall joint health. In this essay, I will discuss practical ways of fortifying your joints at any age.

The first and most important step in fortifying your joints is to maintain a healthy weight. Excess weight can put undue pressure on your joints, especially the knees, hips, and ankles, leading to joint damage. A study conducted by the Journal of Bone and Joint Surgery found that overweight individuals have a higher risk of developing knee osteoarthritis than individuals with a healthy weight. Therefore, it is crucial to maintain a healthy weight by eating a balanced diet and engaging in regular exercise, such as swimming, cycling, or brisk walking.

The second step is to engage in exercises that work the muscles around your joints. Strong muscles help to protect and support your joints, reducing the risk of injury. An article by Harvard Health Publishing recommends engaging in activities such as weightlifting, resistance training, and Pilates. These exercises target specific muscle groups, such as the quadriceps, hamstrings, and calf muscles, which support the knee joints. Furthermore, fitness experts recommend incorporating low-impact exercises, such as yoga and tai chi, which help to improve balance and flexibility.

The third step is to modify your physical activities to reduce stress on your joints. High-impact activities, such as running and jumping, can cause wear and tear on your joints, leading to pain and stiffness. Consider engaging in low-impact activities, such as swimming, cycling, and elliptical training, which provide cardiovascular benefits without putting undue pressure on your joints. If you enjoy running, opt for running shoes with extra cushioning to reduce the impact on your knees, hips, and ankles.

The fourth step is to stretch regularly to improve joint flexibility. Tight muscles can put pressure on your joints, leading to pain and discomfort. A study published by the Journal of Geriatric Physical Therapy found that stretching exercises performed two to three times a week for 12 weeks improved hip range of motion and reduced hip pain in older adults. Consider incorporating static stretching, dynamic stretching, and foam rolling exercises in your workout routine.

The fifth step is to incorporate anti-inflammatory foods in your diet to reduce joint inflammation. Inflammation is a defense mechanism by the body to protect against injury, but chronic inflammation can damage joint tissue, leading to joint pain and stiffness. Foods such as turmeric, ginger, oily fish, nuts, and berries have anti-inflammatory properties and can reduce joint inflammation. Avoid consuming foods high in sugar, saturated fats, and refined carbohydrates, as they can increase the production of inflammatory molecules in the body.

In conclusion, joint health is critical for maintaining an active lifestyle and preventing joint pain and stiffness. Fortifying your joints at any age can reduce the risk of joint injury, slow down the degenerative process, and improve overall joint health. Maintaining a healthy weight, engaging in exercises that work the muscles around your joints, modifying your physical activities to reduce stress on your joints, stretching regularly, and incorporating anti-inflammatory foods in your diet are practical ways of fortifying your joints. By following these steps, you can maintain healthy joints and continue to enjoy an active lifestyle, regardless of your age.

CHAPTER 6

TRAINING SCHEDULE FOR MAXIMUM MUSCLE RECOVERY

Achieving maximum muscle recovery is fundamental in a workout regime for athletes, bodybuilders, and fitness enthusiasts. As the body experiences wear and tear during workouts, proper muscle recovery plays a critical role in repairing the muscles' micro tears and preventing muscle damage. In this essay, we will examine a training schedule that facilitates maximum muscle recovery.

Before delving into the training schedule, it's important to understand what muscle recovery means and why it's necessary. Muscle recovery refers to the process through which the muscles reestablish and regain their strength after a workout. This preliminary restoration after a workout session is vital as it assists the muscle tissue in recovering from the damage that exercise inflicts on the muscle. It helps prevent the inflammation and soreness of muscle tissues and ultimately leads to an increase in overall strength.

One crucial training schedule for maximum muscle recovery entails creating a workout plan that involves two days of rest and five days of intense training. Resting allows the body the necessary time to recuperate and rebuild muscle tissues; while training stimulates muscle fiber growth and improves blood flow. The key to maximum muscle recovery lies in the intensity and frequency of training sessions, as well as the arrangements of rest days.

In the training schedule, the days typically involve an upper-body workout, lower-body workout, and a day of full-body workouts in between the two. A sample workout regimen could include thirty minutes of cardio, followed by an hour-long workout for the specific muscle groups mentioned above. One possible intensity strategy could be to incorporate multijoint exercises that use both your upper and lower body simultaneously, such as squats and lunges.

An ideal plan should avoid working out the same muscle groups on two consecutive days, as this only limits the recovery time necessary for damaged muscles to rejuvenate. Splitting the training regimen with rest days not only allows for muscle recovery but also offers a psychological break, leading to increased motivation and long-term adherence to the program.

To ease muscle discomfort after training, stretching and foam rolling are also worthwhile practices post-workout. Stretching enhances flexibility and improves blood flow to tight muscles, hence increasing the delivery of nutrients and removal of toxins. Foam rolling on the other hand, promotes recovery by both increasing blood flow and decreasing muscle tension. Incorporating these activities in the training schedule further expedites the muscle recovery process.

Diet also plays a critical role in maximum muscle recovery. After workouts, it's essential to consume food that contains carbohydrates and protein. The intake of carbohydrates replenishes the depleted glycogen stores in muscle tissue, and proteins provide the necessary building blocks of amino acids to stimulate muscle growth and reinforce damaged muscle tissue. It's typically advised to refuel within thirty minutes to an hour after exercising as this window of time is when glycogen synthesis is at its highest.

Dehydration impedes a successful muscle recovery process since it makes the body unable to efficiently transport nutrients to the muscle, meaning that adequate hydration is vital. The American Council on Exercise recommends 17-20 ounces of water two-three hours before exercising, and 7-10 oz. every ten to twenty minutes during work out.

In conclusion, maximum muscle recovery is fundamental in any athletic training regime, and a training schedule that brings about this success entails resting for two days in the week and rigorous training for five days. Additionally, incorporating stretching and foam rolling into the training regimen and consuming carbohydrates and proteins within the thirty-minute window post-workout are among the strategies that maximise muscle recovery. Adequate hydration is also a crucial aspect of this training schedule.

CHAPTER 7

HOW TO IDENTIFY AND FIX MUSCLES IMBALANCE

Muscle imbalance is a common issue that can occur when an individual overuses certain muscle groups or neglects others. It can lead to pain, injury, and decreased performance, making it crucial to identify and address any muscle imbalances. In this essay, we will discuss how to identify and fix muscle imbalances.

One way to identify muscle imbalances is to perform a postural assessment. Posture is a key indicator of muscle imbalances, as it can highlight asymmetries and weaknesses in the body. A postural assessment typically involves observing an individual's standing posture from the front, side, and back. Common imbalances that can be identified through a postural assessment include a rounded back, forward head posture, or one shoulder being higher than the other.

A musculoskeletal assessment can also help identify muscle imbalances. This involves testing muscle strength, flexibility, and range of motion to determine if there are any deficits or imbalances present. For example, if an individual has a weak gluteus medius muscle, it can lead to compensatory movement patterns and overuse of other muscles, resulting in an imbalance.

Another way to identify muscle imbalances is to pay attention to what activities or movements cause pain or discomfort. Pain or discomfort during specific movements can indicate muscle imbalances or weaknesses, which need to be addressed. For example, knee pain during a squat can be a sign of weak quadriceps or glute muscles.

Once muscle imbalances have been identified, it is crucial to fix them to prevent further pain or injury. The primary way to fix muscle imbalances is through exercise. This can involve stretches and exercises that target the weaker or underused muscles. Strengthening exercises should be performed with proper form and technique to ensure that the intended muscle is being activated and strengthened.

Stretching is also crucial in addressing muscle imbalances, as it helps to increase flexibility and reduce muscle tension. Stretching the tight or overused muscles can help alleviate pain and correct imbalances. Common stretches for muscle imbalances include hip flexor stretches, chest stretches, and hamstring stretches.

It is important to note that exercise and stretching alone may not fully address muscle imbalances. It may be necessary to seek the guidance of a physical therapist or personal trainer who can create a personalized plan to address the individual's specific imbalances and needs.

In addition to exercise and stretching, other lifestyle factors can contribute to muscle imbalances. Poor posture habits such as prolonged sitting or slouching can lead to imbalances and should be addressed. Adequate rest and recovery are also crucial, as inadequate rest can lead to overuse and muscle strain.

Another factor that can contribute to muscle imbalances is nutrition. Adequate protein intake is essential for muscle repair and growth, while a deficiency in certain vitamins and minerals can lead to muscle weakness. It is crucial to maintain a balanced and nutritious diet to support muscle health.

In conclusion, muscle imbalances can lead to pain, injury, and decreased performance. Identifying and addressing muscle imbalances through exercise, stretching, posture correction, and lifestyle modifications are key to preventing and correcting imbalances. Seeking the guidance of a professional can also be beneficial in creating a personalised plan to address muscle imbalances. With proper attention and care, muscle imbalances can be corrected, leading to improved athletic performance, reduced pain, and enhanced overall health.

CHAPTER 8

HOW TO CORRECT IMBALANCE BONES

Correcting Imbalanced Bones

Bones are an essential part of the body. They provide a framework, give structure and support, and protect our internal organs. However, if bones become imbalanced, it can cause pain and discomfort and lead to more severe health issues. In this essay, I will discuss the causes and solutions for imbalanced bones.

One of the primary causes of imbalanced bones is poor posture. Poor posture can cause one side of the body to bear more weight than the other, leading to uneven wear and tear on the bones. This can cause the spine to curve and tilt, leading to muscle strains, neck pain, back pain, and headaches. Additionally, carrying heavy objects improperly can also cause an imbalance, leading to more stress and strain on the bones.

Another cause of imbalanced bones is injury. If you experience an injury, it can cause misalignments in the bones, leading to an imbalance throughout the body.

Fortunately, there are ways to correct imbalanced bones. One solution is chiropractic care. Chiropractors use spinal manipulation to align and correct imbalanced bones and improve the body's overall function. They use their hands or a specifically designed instrument to apply controlled force to the affected joints, applying pressure to realign them.

Another solution is physical therapy, which focuses on strengthening the affected muscles and improving flexibility. Physical therapy can help relieve pain and correct imbalanced bones by strengthening the muscles and improving posture. Patients will work with specially trained therapists, who will guide them through a series of exercises and stretches, and recommend changes to their daily routine to help improve their overall health.

Massage therapy can also be useful in correcting imbalanced bones. Massage can help to relax muscles and reduce tension and stress in the body. This can ease the pressure on the skeletal system and facilitate proper alignment. Additionally, massage therapy can improve circulation, helping to bring healing nutrients and oxygen to the affected areas.

A healthy diet can also help to correct imbalanced bones. Eating foods rich in calcium and vitamin D, such as milk, yogurt, cheese, and leafy green vegetables, can help to support bone health and strength. Calcium is a critical nutrient that helps to build and support bones, while vitamin D helps the body absorb calcium more effectively.

Another solution is the use of supplements. Supplements such as glucosamine, chondroitin, and omega-3 fatty acids help to protect and support the joints, reducing inflammation, and improving mobility. Consult with a medical professional before taking supplements to ensure safe and effective use.

In conclusion, imbalanced bones can cause pain, discomfort, and restrict mobility. However, there are several solutions available to correct imbalanced bones, including chiropractic care, physical therapy, massage therapy, a healthy diet, and supplements. By taking a proactive approach to bone health, we can decrease our risk of developing severe health issues and maintain optimal function and mobility.

CHAPTER 9

REDUCE FATIGUE

Fatigue, also known as tiredness, is a common symptom experienced by many individuals in their daily lives. It can be a result of physical or mental exertion, lack of sleep, or the presence of an underlying medical condition. In this essay, we will discuss the causes and effects of fatigue, as well as ways to prevent and manage it.

The primary causes of fatigue is as the result for the lack of sleep. A good night's sleep is essential for our bodies to function correctly, and not getting enough sleep can result in daytime fatigue. According to the National Sleep Foundation, adults require between 7-9 hours of sleep per night to feel fully rested and alert. However, many individuals fail to meet this recommended standard, either due to work, familial obligations, or personal activities. This sleep deprivation can lead to daytime drowsiness, irritability, and poor decision-making skills.

Fatigue can also be a symptom of an underlying medical condition. For example, conditions such as anaemia and thyroid disease can lead to fatigue as they cause a decrease in red blood cells and metabolism, respectively. In any instance where fatigue is persistent or accompanied by other symptoms, it is essential to consult a healthcare professional to rule out any underlying medical conditions that may be responsible.

A sedentary lifestyle is another cause of fatigue. Physical activity helps to keep the body alert and energised, and not exercising can cause fatigue. The Centers for Disease Control and Prevention recommends that adults get at least 150 minutes of moderate physical activity weekly to maintain good health. However, many individuals are not physically active enough, leading to a lack of energy and alertness. Incorporating regular physical activity into our daily routine can help prevent fatigue.

Moreover, many lifestyle factors can exacerbate fatigue. For example, excessive caffeine consumption and smoking can both lead to fatigue. While caffeine may provide temporary energy boosts, consuming too much can lead to insomnia and other sleep-related issues, exacerbating fatigue. Similarly, smoking can lead to poor circulation, respiratory issues, and reduced oxygen uptake, all of which can lead to fatigue.

The detrimental effects of fatigue are far-reaching. One of the primary effects is reduced productivity. When we are fatigued, it becomes more challenging to focus, make decisions, and complete tasks. The reduced performance is not just limited to cognitive tasks. Individuals experiencing fatigue may also perform poorly in physical tasks, causing accidents and injuries.

Additionally, fatigue can also have an impact on our mental and emotional health. When we are tired, we may experience anxiety, depression, and reduced attention span. These effects can lead to decreased motivation and an overall sense of apathy.

Preventing fatigue is the key to achieving better overall health. Incorporating regular exercise into our daily routine, maintaining a healthy diet, and getting enough sleep are all important ways to prevent fatigue. Additionally, reducing consumption of caffeine and alcohol and quitting smoking are essential elements in preventing fatigue and maintaining good health.

In conclusion, fatigue is a common symptom that can arise due to several different causes. Lack of sleep, underlying medical conditions, a sedentary lifestyle, excessive caffeine and alcohol consumption, and smoking all contribute to fatigue. The effects of fatigue are far-reaching, including reduced productivity, physical accidents, as well as mental and emotional health issues. Preventing fatigue requires maintaining a healthy lifestyle, including exercise, healthy eating habits, and getting enough sleep. Identifying the cause of fatigue and seeking medical assistance when necessary is also imperative in managing fatigue.

CHAPTER 10

CREATE GREATER LUNGS CAPACITY

Creating Greater Lung Capacity: An Essential Aspect of Physical Health

Lung capacity refers to the maximum amount of air that a person can inhale and exhale during peaceful breathing. Lung capacity is a crucial factor that determines the overall health of an individual. Poor lung capacity has adverse effects on the body, such as shortness of breath, fatigue, and weakened immune function. Moreover, individuals with poor lung capacity are at higher risk of developing lung diseases such as asthma and chronic obstructive pulmonary disease (COPD). Therefore, it is imperative for individuals to strive to improve their lung capacity to enhance their overall health and quality of life. This essay focuses on ways to create greater lung capacity, including regular physical activity, breathing exercises and avoiding smoking.

One of the most effective ways of increasing lung capacity is by engaging in regular physical activity such as cardio exercises. Numerous studies have revealed a strong correlation between physical activity and lung capacity. Various forms of physical activity, such as running, jogging, cycling or brisk walking have been shown to have a positive effect on lung capacity. One study conducted by Johnson et al., (2018) found that runners had a higher lung capacity and less respiratory abnormalities than non-runners. Similarly, a study by Kampert et al., (2019) showed that engaging in regular physical activity significantly increased lung capacity, particularly in individuals who were initially sedentary. These findings indicate that physical activity is essential in increasing lung capacity, and individuals should incorporate regular exercise in their daily routine.

In addition to physical activity, engaging in breathing exercises like pranayama poses can help improve lung capacity. Pranayama poses are breathing exercises aimed at increasing lung volume and oxygen intake. These exercises involve inhaling slowly and deeply and exhaling slowly while counting the number of seconds. A study by Tyagi et al., (2018) showed that individuals who engaged in pranayama exercises had significantly improved lung capacity, with an increase in the volume of air exchanged during breathing. The study highlighted the importance of breathing exercises as a natural and non-invasive way to improve lung capacity.

Apart from engaging in physical exercises and breathing exercises, avoiding smoking can help create greater lung capacity. Smoking is a significant contributor to respiratory problems, including lung cancer, COPD, and poor lung function. Cigarette smoke contains harmful chemicals that can irritate and damage the lungs, leading to decreased lung function. According to the American Lung Association (2019), smokers tend to have a lower lung capacity than non-smokers, with long-term consequences on their health. Quitting smoking can help improve lung capacity and reduce the risk of developing respiratory problems. However, it is essential to note that quitting smoking is a challenging process and may require several attempts before settling successfully.

In conclusion, lung capacity is an essential aspect of overall health, and individuals should strive to improve it. Regular physical activity such as cardio exercises, pranayama breathing exercises, and avoiding smoking can help create greater lung capacity and enhance overall health. Although improving lung capacity may not be easy and may take time, the benefits, such as an increase in energy levels and reduced risk of respiratory problems, are worth the effort. It is essential to consult a qualified healthcare provider before starting any exercise routine or breathing exercises to determine the best course of action.

CHAPTER 11

ENHANCE THE EFFECTIVENESS OF MEDICATIONS

Enhancing the Effectiveness of Medications on Your Body

Medications are an integral part of healthcare. They are used to treat a wide variety of conditions ranging from minor illnesses to life-threatening diseases. When you take these medications, you expect them to work effectively and quickly. However, this is not always the case. Sometimes medications do not work as fast or as well as we expect them to. This can be due to a variety of reasons, including our body's response to the medication, or the way we take the medication. In this essay, we will discuss some of the ways in which we can enhance the effectiveness of medications on our body.

The first step in enhancing the effectiveness of medication is to understand how the medication works and what it does in the body. Once you have this knowledge, you can take the medication as prescribed, and in the right dose. This is important because taking too much or too little of the medication can lead to adverse effects or the medication not being effective. For example, if you are prescribed an antibiotic to treat an infection, it is important to take the full course of the medication, as prescribed, even if you start to feel better after a few days. This is because stopping the medication too soon can lead to the infection returning, often in a more severe form.

Another important factor to consider when taking medication is the timing of the dose. Some medications work best when taken at specific times of the day. For example, some medications are best taken in the morning, while others are best taken in the evening, or before bedtime. This is because the medication's effectiveness is influenced by the body's natural rhythms, or circadian rhythms. Circadian rhythms are the internal biological clock that regulates various physiological processes in the body, including sleep-wake cycles, hormone production, and metabolism. Therefore, taking medication at specific times can improve its effectiveness.

In addition to the timing of the medication, the way the medication is taken can also affect its effectiveness. For example, some medications are best taken with food, while others are best taken on an empty stomach. This is because food can affect the absorption of the medication into the body. Similarly, some medications are best swallowed whole, while others can be crushed or dissolved in water. The method of administration can also affect the medication's effectiveness. For example, some medications are intended to be injected, while others are intended to be inhaled or applied topically. Understanding how to take medication correctly can improve the medication's effectiveness.

It is also important to consider other factors that can affect the medication's effectiveness. For example, smoking cigarettes can affect the absorption of some medications and reduce their effectiveness. Therefore, it is recommended that you try to quit smoking or reduce your tobacco intake if you are taking medication. Similarly, drinking alcohol can also affect the absorption and metabolism of medication, and reduce its effectiveness. Therefore, it is recommended that you avoid alcohol when taking medication.

Another way to enhance the effectiveness of medication is to pay attention to your overall health and wellbeing. This includes eating a healthy diet, getting regular exercise, and reducing stress. Good health can improve the body's ability to absorb and metabolise medication, which can enhance its effectiveness. Exercise, in particular, can improve blood flow and increase the absorption of medication into the body. Reducing stress can also improve the body's ability to metabolise medication by reducing stress hormones that can interfere with the medication's effectiveness.

In conclusion, medications are an essential part of healthcare, but their effectiveness can be influenced by various factors. Understanding how medication works and how to take it correctly can improve its effectiveness. Paying attention to timing, the method of administration, and other factors that can affect effectiveness,such as smoking and alcohol consumption,can also improve medication effectiveness. Furthermore, maintaining good health and reducing stress can enhance the body's ability to absorb and metabolise medication, improving its effectiveness. By following these guidelines, we can enhance the effectiveness of medication and improve our health and wellbeing.

CHAPTER 12

RHEUMATOID ARTHRITIS

Rheumatoid arthritis(RA) is a habitual autoimmune complaint that affects roughly 1% of the global population, with an advanced frequency in women and aged individuals. The complaint primarily targets the synovial joints, ultimately leading to cartilage and bone corrosion, common disfigurement, and disability if left undressed. The exact causes of RA aren't completely understood, but experimenters believe that genetics, environmental factors, and dysregulation of the vulnerable system play a part. The hallmark point of RA is common pain, swelling, stiffness, and tenderheartedness that affect both sides of the body and persist for further than six weeks. The symptoms generally start in the small joints of the hands and bases, but they can also occur in the wrists, elbows, shoulders, hips, knees, and ankles. As RA progresses, the joints lose their inflexibility and range of stir, making it delicate to perform diurnal conditioning similar as grasping, codifying, walking, and climbing stairs. piecemeal from the joints, RA can also affect other organs and systems in the body, causing a range of complications. For illustration, RA cases may witness inflammation of the eyes, lung, heart, and blood vessels, which can lead to vision loss, respiratory failure, cardiovascular complaint, and anaemia. also, RA cases have an increased threat of developing osteoporosis, depression, fatigue, and weight loss, which can further reduce their quality of life. The croaker will estimate the case's symptoms, medical history, and physical findings, similar as common tenderheartedness, swelling, and disfigurement. The croaker will also order blood tests to assess the position of seditious labels, antibodies, and other factors that are specific to RA, similar as rheumatoid factor and anti-cyclic citrullinated peptide(anti-CCP) antibodies. Eventually, the croaker may perform imaging studies similar asX-rays, ultrasound, or glamorous resonance imaging(MRI) to estimate the extent of common damage and complaint exertion. Although there's presently no cure for RA, several treatment options are available to palliate the symptoms, decelerate down the complaint progression, and help complications. The most common treatments include non-steroidal anti-inflammatory medicines(NSAIDs), complaint- modifying anti-rheumatic medicines(DMARDs), birth agents, and corticosteroids. NSAIDs are useful for relieving pain and inflammation in the short term, but they've limited goods on the underpinning complaint. DMARDs, on the other hand, work by targeting the vulnerable system and reducing the exertion of seditious cells, thereby decelerating down the damage to the joints. Birth agents are a newer class of specifics that block specific motes involved in the seditious process, similar as tumour necrosis factor(TNF) or interleukins(ILs). These agents can be more effective than traditional DMARDs in some cases, but they also carry a advanced threat of adverse goods, similar as infections and malice. Corticosteroids, similar as prednisone, are important anti-inflammatory medicines that can fleetly reduce the symptoms of RA, but they also have significant side goods over the long term, similar as weight gain, diabetes, and osteoporosis. In addition to drug, RA cases can also profit from non-pharmacologic interventions that target common mobility, strength, and function. These interventions include physical remedy, occupational remedy, and exercise programs acclimatised to the case's requirements and capacities. Physical remedy involves the use of homemade ways, heat remedy, cold remedy, and electrical stimulation to relieve pain and ameliorate common inflexibility. Occupational remedy focuses on tutoring the case how to perform diurnal conditioning with lower stress on the joints, similar as using adaptive bias, modifying home and plant surroundings, and learning energy-conservation ways. Exercise programs, similar to calisthenics, range- of- stir exercises, and strength training, can help ameliorate common health, reduce inflammation, and enhance overall well- being. In conclusion, rheumatoid arthritis is a habitual autoimmune complaint that affects millions of people worldwide and can lead to common damage, disability, and other complications if not treated duly. The complaint is characterised by common pain, swelling, stiffness, and tenderheartedness, and can also affect other organs and systems in the body. While there's no

cure for RA, several treatment options are available that can palliate the symptoms and decelerate down the complaint progression, similar as NSAIDs, DMARDs,birth————————- ——————————
-agents,and
corticosteroids.Inaddition,non-pharmacologic interventions similarphysical remedy, occupational remedy, and exercise programs can also be salutary for RA cases. With the right combination of treatments, RA cases can achieve better quality of life and maintain their functional independence for longer.

WAYS TO PREVENT RHEUMATOID ARTHRITIS

Rheumatoid arthritis(RA) is a habitual autoimmune complaint that causes common inflammation and damage. RA affects about 1.3 million Americans and can lead to severe disability if not managed metly. Although there's no sure way to help RA, there are certain life changes that people can make to reduce their threat of developing this complaint. One of the most critical ways to help RA is to maintain a healthy weight. People who are fat or fat are at an advanced threat of developing RA than those who maintain a healthy weight. The redundant weight puts added pressure on the joints, making them more susceptible to damage. To maintain a healthy weight, people should eat a balanced diet with plenty of fruits and vegetables, whole grains, and spare protein sources. They should also limit their input of impregnated and trans fats, added sugars, and reused foods. Regular exercise is also essential for maintaining a healthy weight and reducing the threat of RA. Exercise helps to make strong muscles and bones, ameliorate common inflexibility and range of stir, and reduce inflammation throughout the body. Another critical factor in precluding RA is to avoid or quit smoking. Studies have shown that smoking is a significant threat factor for developing RA, and it can also worsen the symptoms of RA in people who formerly have the complaint. Smoking triggers an autoimmune response in the body, which can lead to habitual inflammation and common damage. Quitting smoking is the stylish option for your health. Talk to your croaker about ways to quit smoking, similar to nicotine relief remedy or tradition specifics. Maintaining good oral hygiene is also essential for precluding RA. Recent studies have shown a link between good complaints and an increased threat of RA. The bacteria that beget good complaints can enter the bloodstream and spark an vulnerable response that can lead to habitual inflammation throughout the body, including the joints. To reduce the threat of good complaints, people should brush and floss their teeth regularly, and visit the dentist for regular cleanings and checks. Reducing stress is another critical step in precluding RA. Stress can weaken the vulnerable system and detector inflammation throughout the body, including the joints. To reduce stress, people should exercise relaxation ways similar to deep breathing, contemplation, or yoga. They should also identify the sources of stress in their lives and find ways to avoid or manage them. In addition to these life changes, there are also some vitamins and supplements that may help reduce the threat of RA. For illustration, vitamin D plays a pivotal part in maintaining bone health and may also help reduce inflammation throughout the body. People can get vitamin D naturally from the sun or through foods similar to adipose fish and fortified dairy products. Supplements are also available if demanded. Omega- 3 adipose acids, which are set up in fish oil painting, may also help reduce inflammation in people with RA. Still, further exploration is demanded to confirm the benefits of these supplements for precluding RA. In conclusion, there are several life changes that people can make to reduce their threat of developing RA. Maintaining a healthy weight, quitting smoking, maintaining good oral hygiene, reducing stress, and taking vitamins and supplements may all help reduce the threat of RA. By making these changes, individualities can take control of their health and reduce their threat of developing this enervating complaint.

FOOD THAT CAUSES RHEUMATOID ARTHRITIS

As rheumatoid arthritis(RA) affects millions of people worldwide, it's pivotal to examine the implicit causes of this autoimmune complaint duly. Although RA has multifactorial causes, some studies suggest that certain foods might complicate the inflammation and contribute to its development. Thus, in this essay, I'll describe some common foods that might beget or worsen rheumatoid arthritis and examine the scientific substantiation behind these claims.   Originally, let's explore the role of red meat in RA development. Some studies argue that consuming high quantities of red meat might increase the threat of developing rheumatoid arthritis. This proposition is grounded on the fact that red meat contains a type of protein called Neu5Gc, which our bodies can not produce naturally. As a result, when we eat red meat, our vulnerable system recognizes Neu5Gc as foreign and triggers an seditious response to exclude it. Still, this response can occasionally lead to habitual inflammation, which is a given cause of RA development. Also, red meat is high in arachidonic acid, an omega-6 adipose acid that can promote inflammation when not balanced with enough omega- 3 adipose acids. Thus, some scientists believe that reducing red meat input might palliate the symptoms of RA and lower the threat of its development.   Secondly, let's explore the implicit link between gluten and RA. Gluten is a type of protein set up in wheat, barley, and rye, and some people might have an inheritable predilection to gluten perceptivity, known as celiac complaint. Still, indeed people without celiac complaints can have a gluten dogmatism or perceptivity, which might manifest as colourful symptoms, including common pain and inflammation. Thus, some studies suggest that barring gluten from the diet might ameliorate the symptoms of RA and reduce the threat of developing it. In fact, a small study published in the Journal of Nutrition and Metabolism set up that RA cases who followed a gluten-free diet for one time had significant reductions in pain, common stiffness, and inflammation labels compared to the control group. Still, further exploration is demanded to confirm this link and determine the optimal gluten input for RA cases. Incidentally, let's bandy the implicit damages of vegetable canvases in RA cases. Vegetable canvases , similar to sludge, sunflower, soybean, and safflower canvases , contain high quantities of omega- 6 adipose acids and low quantities of omega- 3 adipose acids. As mentioned before, omega- 6 adipose acids can promote inflammation when not balanced with enough omega- 3 adipose acids, which might worsen the symptoms of RA. Also, some vegetable canvases might contain trans fats, which are known to be dangerous to mortal health and might promote inflammation and oxidative stress. Thus, some scientists suggest that reducing the input of vegetable canvases might ameliorate the symptoms of RA and help its progression. Rather, they recommend using healthier canvases with a balanced omega- 3 to omega- 6 rate, similar to olive oil painting, avocado oil painting, or coconut oil painting. In conclusion, while the causes of rheumatoid arthritis are complex and multifaceted, some substantiation suggests that specific foods might affect its development and progression. Red meat, gluten, and vegetable canvases are three common suspects that might complicate inflammation and joint pain in RA cases. Still, further exploration is demanded to confirm these links and determine the optimal salutary strategy for RA cases. Thus, if you have RA or know someone who does, it's essential to consult a medical professional or a registered dietitian for personalised advice and treatment. By following a well-balanced and nutrient- thick diet, avoiding eventuality triggers, and staying physically active, RA cases can manage their symptoms and ameliorate their quality of life.

FOOD THAT HELP IN REDUCING RHEUMATOID ARTHRITIS

Rheumatoid arthritis is known as an autoimmune complaint that causes inflammation in the joints. inflammation turns to pain, swelling, and stiffness. While there is no cure for rheumatoid arthritis, making salutary changes is one way to help manage the symptoms. Certain foods have been shown to reduce inflammation and promote overall common health, while others have the contrary effect. In this essay, we will bandy the foods that can help reduce rheumatoid arthritis symptoms. First on the list is fish. Fish is a great source of omega- 3 adipose acids, which have been shown to reduce inflammation in the body. In fact, a study published in the Journal of the American College of Nutrition set up that omega- 3 supplements reduced common pain and stiffness in rheumatoid arthritis cases. Eating fish regularly can give the same benefits as taking supplements, as well as furnishing other important vitamins and minerals. Some great examples of fish that are high in omega- 3s include tuna, and mackerel.   Another great food for reducing rheumatoid arthritis symptoms is fruits and vegeta. They also contain other important vitamins and minerals that support   common health. A study published in the journal Arthritis Research and Therapy set up that a diet rich in fruits and vegetables was associated with a lower threat of developing rheumatoid arthritis. Some great   exemplifications of fruits and vegetables to include in your diet are berrie, and lush flora.   Nuts and seeds are another great food to include in your diet if you suffer from rheumatoid arthritis. They're high in omega- 3 adipose acids and antioxidants, which help to reduce inflammation in the body. A study published in the Journal of Nutrition set up that eating nuts and seeds regularly was associated with a lower threat of developing   rheumatoid   arthritis.   Some   great exemplifications of nuts and seeds to include in your diet are almonds, walnuts, and chia seeds.   Spices and sauces are also great for reducing inflammation in the body. Turmeric, in particular, has been shown to be an effective anti-inflammatory. A study published in the journal Phytotherapy Research set up that turmeric reduced   common pain and swelling in rheumatoid arthritis cases. A study published in the Journal of Medicinal Food set up that gusto reduces inflammation in the body and improves   common mobility in rheumatoid arthritis cases.   Eventually, it's important to avoid foods that can beget inflammation in the body. This includes reused and fried foods, red meat, and ameliorated carbohydrates. These foods can lead to inflammation   and   complicate   the   symptoms   of rheumatoid arthritis. In conclusion, there are numerous foods that can help reduce the symptoms of rheumatoid arthritis. Fish, fruits and vegetables, nuts and seeds, and spices and sauces are each great options to include in your diet. By making salutary changes and avoiding seditious foods, you can help manage the symptoms of rheumatoid arthritis and ameliorate your overall quality of life.

CHAPTER 13

OSTEOARTHRITIS

Osteoarthritis is a medical condition that affects millions of people worldwide, particularly those over the age of 60. It's a type of arthritis that occurs when the cartilage between bones starts to deteriorate, leading to pain and stiffness in the joints. Although osteoarthritis is frequently associated with ageing, it can also be caused by injury or other underpinning medical conditions. It's a habitual condition that can oppressively impact an existent's mobility and quality of life. In this essay, we will bandy the causes, symptoms, and treatment options for osteoarthritis. One of the main causes of osteoarthritis is the natural wear and tear and gash of the joints over time. As we progress, the cartilage between our bones begins to break down, leading to disunion and inflammation in the joints. This can beget significant discomfort, particularly in weight- bearing joints similar to the hips and knees. Still, osteoarthritis can also be caused by injury or trauma to the joints, infection, or common abnormalities. In some cases, genetics may also play a part in an existent's liability of developing osteoarthritis.The symptoms of osteoarthritis can vary from person to person but generally include pain and stiffness in the affected joint. Other symptoms may include swelling, tenderheartedness, or a grating sensation when moving the joint. The symptoms may worsen over time, and as the condition progresses, individualities may witness a limited range of stir in the affected areas, Just as walking or standing for lord ages. In severe cases, osteoarthritis can lead to disability and may bear surgical intervention. There are several treatment options available for osteoarthritis, ranging from life changes to drug and surgical procedures. One of the most effective ways to manage osteoarthritis is through exercise and weight operation. Exercise can help ameliorate common mobility and reduce pain and stiffness, while weight operation can help reduce the cargo on weight- bearing joints. Physical remedy may also be recommended to help individuals develop an acclimatized exercise program that's safe and effective for their condition.   In addition to exercise and weight operation, drug can also be used to manage the symptoms. In severe cases, surgical procedures similar to common relief surgery may be necessary to restore common function and mobility.   It's important to note that while there's no cure for osteoarthritis, early intervention and operation can significantly ameliorate an existent's quality of life. Regular check- ups with a healthcare provider can help ensure that the condition is duly managed, and treatment options can be acclimated as demanded. Also, individuals with osteoarthritis should be encouraged to maintain a healthy life, including regular exercise, healthy eating habits, and stress operation practices. In conclusion, osteoarthritis is a common condition that can significantly impact an existent's mobility and quality of life. While there's no cure for osteoarthritis, early intervention and operation can help individuals more manage their symptoms and ameliorate their overall health. Treatment options range from life changes to drug and surgical procedures, and individualities should work nearly with their healthcare providers to develop an acclimatized treatment plan. With the right operation and support, individualities with osteoarthritis can still lead fulfilling and active lives.

CAUSES OF OSTEOARTHRITIS

Osteoarthritis, also known as degenerative common complaint, is a condition that affects millions of people around the world. It's a common cause of disability, especially among aged grown- ups. In osteoarthritis, the cartilage that cocoons the ends of bones in joints begins to break down and wear down. This can beget pain, stiffness, and loss of mobility. The causes of osteoarthritis are not fully understood, but multitudinous factors are known to contribute to its development. One of the main causes of osteoarthritis is growing. As we get aged, the cartilage in our joints begins to deteriorate. This can beget the bones to rub against each other, leading to pain and inflammation. Another major cause of osteoarthritis is genetics. Studies have shown that certain genes can increase a person's trouble of developing the condition. For illustration, a gene called GDF5 has been linked to an increased trouble of osteoarthritis in the knee. obesity and being fat can also contribute to the development of osteoarthritis. spare weight can put spare stress on the joints, causing the cartilage to wear down more snappily. This can lead to osteoarthritis in weight- bearing joints like the knees and hips. Injuries and overuse of joints can also lead to osteoarthritis. Athletes and people who engage in repetitive movements like codifying or using a computer mouse are at particular trouble for developing the condition. Injuries to joints can damage the cartilage and lead to osteoarthritis subsequently in life. Other factors that may contribute to the development of osteoarthritis include gender(women are more likely to develop the condition than men), bone scars, and experimental conditions like hip dysplasia. While the exact causes of osteoarthritis are not fully understood, there are some way individualities can take to reduce their trouble of developing the condition. Maintaining a healthy weight through diet and exercise can help reduce stress on the joints and help devilish wear and tear and gash and incision. Engaging in regular physical exertion can also help strengthen the muscles around the joints, furnishing fresh support. Avoiding injuries to the joints is important as well. Athletes and people who engage in repetitive movements should take way to cover their joints from damage. This may include wearing protective gear or taking frequent breaks from repetitive exertion. There is no cure for osteoarthritis, but there are treatments available to help manage symptoms. Pain relievers, analogous as acetaminophen or nonsteroidalanti- seditious drugs(NSAIDs), can help reduce pain and inflammation. Physical remedy and exercise can also be effective in perfecting mobility and reducing pain. In some cases, common relief surgery may be necessary. In conclusion, osteoarthritis is a common cause of disability and can be caused by a combination of factors including aging, genetics, obesity, injuries, and overuse of joints. While there is no cure for the condition, there are way individualities can take to reduce their trouble of developing it and treatments available to manage symptoms. recognizing the trouble factors and taking preventative measures can go a long way in maintaining common health and preventing the onset of osteoarthritis.

PREVENTION OF OSTEOARTHRITIS

Osteoarthritis is a degenerative common complaint that generally affects the elderly but can also impact youthful individualities. It's the most common form of arthritis, counting for over 80 of all cases. The condition is characterised by the breakdown of cartilage, which leads to pain and stiffness in the joints. While there is no cure for osteoarthritis, there are several approaches to help the progression of the complaint. Prevention of osteoarthritis starts beforehand, indeed before symptoms appear. Some of the swish ways to help osteoarthritis include maintaining a healthy weight and exercise regularly. spare weight places a significant amount of stress on the joints, particularly the hips, knees, and back. In addition, weight operation lowers a person's trouble of other habitual conditions, including heart complaint, diabetes, and cancer. Regular exercise, particularly strength training exercises, can help maintain common strictness, muscle strength, and balance. Another pivotal preventative strategy is to maintain good common health by avoiding overuse or injury. Athletes, in particular, should exercise proper fashion and use proper outfit to avoid stressing the joints excessively. individualities who partake in high- impact sports analogous as soccer and basketball, may also want to consider using knee pads or other protective outfit to reduce the trouble of common injury. Diet also plays an important part in preventing osteoarthritis. A diet rich in fruits, vegetables, and whole grains has been shown to help reduce inflammation that can lead to common pain and stiffness. In- seditious foods analogous as adipose fish, nuts, and seeds may offer fresh protection against the condition. Again, diets high in saturated fat, perfected carbohydrates, and sugar may increase the trouble of developing osteoarthritis. In recent times, several necessary antidotes have surfaced as implicit preventative options for osteoarthritis. For illustration, acupuncture has been used to help palliate common pain and reduce inflammation in the body. Physical remedy, massage, and chiropractic care may also give relief for individualities with osteoarthritis symptoms. still, it's important to flash back that the effectiveness of these antidotes varies considerably, and individualities should consult with their providers before beginning any new treatment. In addition to life changes and necessary antidotes, several specifics can help help the progression of osteoarthritis. Nonsteroidalanti- seditious drugs(NSAIDs) analogous as ibuprofen can help reduce inflammation, while corticosteroids can help relieve pain and swelling in the joints. further recently, injections of hyaluronic acid have been used to help gyroplane the joints and reduce disunion between the bones, furnishing temporary relief for individualities with osteoarthritis. The key to preventing osteoarthritis is early intervention. While there is no cure for the condition, a combination of life changes, necessary antidotes, and medicine can help delay or indeed help the progression of the complaint. also, close monitoring by a healthcare provider can help descry and treat symptoms before they come severe. In conclusion, osteoarthritis is a enervating condition that can significantly impact an existent's quality of life. still, there are several preventative measures that can help brake or indeed help its progression. Maintaining a healthy weight, exercising regularly, and avoiding overuse or injury are just a numerous ways to help osteoarthritis. also, those who are at high trouble for osteoarthritis should consider necessary antidotes and medicine to help manage the condition. With proper operation and care, individualities can maintain common health and enjoy an active, pain-free life for times to come.

PREVALENCE FOR OSTEOARTHRITIS

Osteoarthritis is a habitual, progressive complaint of the joints which results in the degeneration of cartilage and growth of new bone in and around the joints. It's one of the most common common conditions worldwide, which majorly affects the elderly population.

Osteoarthritis is associated with various trouble factors that include aging, obesity, common injury, occupation or sports, and heritable partiality. The frequency of osteoarthritis is adding worldwide, and it's estimated that roughly 10 of the population progressed above 60 times suffers from this condition. According to the World Health Organization(WHO), roughly 80 of people with osteoarthritis have limitations in movement, and 25 can't perform their quotidian exertion of living. likewise, it's noteworthy that osteoarthritis is the alternate most common cause of disability in the elderly population after cardiovascular conditions. Several studies have been conducted on the frequency of osteoarthritis. In one of the studies conducted, the data from the National Health and Nutrition Examination Survey(NHANES) revealed that the frequency of osteoarthritis in the United States increased from6.6 in 1999 to9.0 in 2014. This increase in frequency is associated with an increase in obesity and growing population. The study further reported that osteoarthritis was more current in ladies(10.5) than males(6.7) in both these time frames. Another study compared the frequency of osteoarthritis in different countries. The study reported that knee osteoarthritis was more common in former Soviet republic as compared to other countries. likewise, the frequency of osteoarthritis is also high in Australia, Europe, and Asia, with middle-aged to elderly people being the most affected. The frequence of osteoarthritis in women is also advanced than in men, especially after menopause when the product of estrogen declines in women. Several trouble factors are responsible for the increased frequency of osteoarthritis. Aging is the foremost trouble factor which affects the quality and volume of cartilage. Aging also causes common instability and declination of the menisci and ligaments, leading to osteoarthritis. obesity is another significant trouble factor, which can be related to increased mechanical stress on weight- bearing joints, particularly the hip and knee joints. also, common injury or surgery can also lead to osteoarthritis, and it can be due to the development ofpost- traumatic osteoarthritis. Sports exertion, analogous as running or football, also enhance the trouble of developing osteoarthritis. There are various treatment options available for osteoarthritis, including nonpharmacological, pharmacological, and surgical interventions. Nonpharmacological interventions include exercise, weight loss, and the use of walking aids, whereas pharmacological interventions include the use of nonsteroidalanti- seditious drugs(NSAIDs), anesthetics, and other characteristic treatments. Surgical interventions include common relief surgery which is an effective and long- standing treatment for end- stage osteoarthritis, especially of the hip and knee joints. In conclusion, osteoarthritis is a current common complaint that ultimately affects the elderly population. The frequence of osteoarthritis is adding worldwide, and it's one of the leading causes of disability in the elderly population. The high frequency of osteoarthritis is related to various trouble factors like growing, obesity, common injury, occupation or sports, and heritable factors. The effective operation of osteoarthritis generally requires a combination of nonpharmacologic and pharmacologic interventions. still, common relief surgery remains the only treatment option for advanced stages of osteoarthritis.

CHAPTER 14

SMART EXERCISES FOR PEOPLE WITH ANKYLOSING SPONDYLITIS

Ankylosing spondylitis(AS) is a habitual inflammatory complaint that primarily affects the spine and sacroiliac joints. It leads to pain and stiffness in the rear, which can eventually beget a stooped posture. An optimal approach to managing AS involves a combination of medicine and exercise. Exercise, in particular, plays a vital part in perfecting common mobility, reducing pain, preventing complications, and enhancing overall physical and internal health. still, not all exercises are created equal. Smart exercise is necessary for people with AS to ensure the maximum benefits with minimal detriment. Smart exercise for AS involves a balance between two primary objects- perfecting strictness and strengthening muscles. Stretching exercises aim to increase the range of stir of affected joints, help scars, and meliorate posture. Strengthening exercises, on the other hand, aim to increase muscle strength and abidance, which, in turn, stabilizes affected joints and reduces pain. One of the most effective stretching exercises for AS is the McKenzie extension exercise. It involves lying face down on the bottom and propping up on your elbows, gently arching your lower rear. This exercise is useful in perfecting spinal extension, reducing pain, and preventing scars. Another stretching exercise that could be salutary for people with AS is the casket expansion exercise. It involves standing in a doorway and pushing your arms against the doorway frame, stretching your casket muscles and perfecting overall posture. Strengthening exercises for AS must concentrate on the muscles that support the spine, analogous as the abdominal, back, and hip muscles. Bridging exercises, which involve lying on the rear and raising the hips off the bottom, can strengthen the glutes, hamstrings, and lower rear muscles, which help stabilise the spine. also, planks, which involve holding the body in a straight line parallel to the bottom, can strengthen the abdominal and back muscles. These exercises are low- impact and help reduce the strain on affected joints. Cardiovascular exercise, analogous as brisk walking, cycling, or swimming, can meliorate overall fitness and health, aid in weight operation, reduce inflammation, and meliorate common mobility. still, it's essential to choose the right intensity, duration, and type of exercise to avoid driving a flare- up. It's rather a low- impact exercise, analogous as cycling, that does not complicate the symptoms but provides respectable cardiovascular benefit. An important consideration while choosing exercises for AS is to avoid high- impact exertion analogous as jogging, running, or jumping, which can beget microtrauma to the joints, leading to inflammation and pain. also, exercises that involve twisting, bending forward, or heavy lifting can lead to spinal fractures and should be avoided. It's vital to hear to your body and be alive of any signs of pain, discomfort, or fatigue. Starting with low- intensity exercises and gradually adding the intensity and duration over time can help minimise the trouble of injury and maximise the benefits. In conclusion, smart exercise is a vital element of the operation of AS, helping to meliorate common mobility, reduce pain, help complications, and promote overall physical and internal health. A balanced approach that includes stretching, strengthening, and cardiovascular exercises can give maximum benefits with minimum detriment. It's critical to choose the right type, duration, and intensity of exercise, keeping in mind individual conditions, preferences, and limitations. By incorporating smart exercise into quotidian routines, people with AS can take an active part in managing their condition and enhancing their quality of life.

CHAPTER 15

BEST SLEEPING POSITION FOR PEOPLE WITH ANKYLOSING SPONDYLITIS

Ankylosing spondylitis(AS) is a habitual condition that primarily affects the spine, performing in inflammation, pain, and stiffness. People with AS constantly struggle to find a comfortable sleeping position due to the nature of the complaint. Chancing the swish resting position can help reduce pain and discomfort, ultimately leading to better rest. In this essay, we will bat the swish resting positions for people with ankylosing spondylitis. The first resting position that can benefit people with ankylosing spondylitis is sleeping on your reverse. This position helps maintain the natural wind of the spine and reduces pressure on the joints. Placing a pillow under the knees can give further support and ease pressure on the lower reverse. still, people with AS who substantiation breathing difficulties while sleeping should avoid sleeping on their rear as it can worsen the symptoms. also, those who snuffle loudly should avoid this position too as it increases the snoring. The alternate resting position that can be helpful for people with AS is sleeping on the side. Sleeping on the side with a pillow between the knees can give fresh support and reduce the pressure on the lower reverse. It's important to choose the right pillow while sleeping in this position to help shoulder and neck pain. AS cases should avoid sleeping on the same side for an extended period and alternate sides to help discomfort and pressure points. The third resting position that is constantly recommended for people with AS is sleeping on the stomach. While this position can be salutary for those floundering with sleep apnea, it is not a recommended position for people with ankylosing spondylitis. Sleeping on the stomach can beget the spine to strain and stress the muscles, leading to discomfort and pain. therefore, it's swish to avoid this position if you have AS. In conclusion, chancing the right resting position is vital for people with ankylosing spondylitis to reduce pain and meliorate the quality of their sleep. Sleeping on your rear with a pillow under the knees, sleeping on the side with a pillow between the knees, or choosing a supportive mattress and pillow can help give relief and comfort. still, it's essential to choose a position that suits your individual conditions and to consult with a croaker or physical therapist before trying any new resting positions.

CHAPTER 16

THINGS WOMEN WITH ANKYLOSING SPONDYLITIS NEED TO KNOW

Ankylosing Spondylitis affects the spine. AS can also affect other joints and organs in the body, analogous as the eyes, heart, and lungs. Anyone can develop AS, but it's more common in men than women. still, women with AS constantly face unique challenges that they need to be alive of in order to more manage their condition. One important thing that women with AS need to know is the impact that the complaint can have on their reproductive health. Studies have shown that AS can increase the trouble of premature birth, low birth weight, and complications during gravidity. also, women with AS may have difficulty conceiving or carrying a gravidity to term. They should bat their options with their healthcare provider to ensure they admit the swish care for themselves and their future children. Another critical aspect of AS that women should understand is the impact on bone health. AS causes inflammation that can lead to bone loss, putting women at increased trouble for osteoporosis. Women with AS should speak with their healthcare providers about regular bone-density testing and strategies for maintaining bone health, analogous as weight- bearing exercises, calcium and vitamin D input, and medicine if necessary. Women with AS also need to be alive of the impact of their complaint on their emotional good. Due to the habitual pain and limited mobility that AS can beget, women with the complaint are at trouble for depression and anxiety. They should not stagger to speak with their healthcare provider or a internal health professional if they notice changes in their mood or if they feel overwhelmed by their condition. One fresh challenge that women with AS may face in their quotidian lives is chancing comfortable vesture that accommodates their common pain and stiffness. multitudinous women with AS find that looser, springy fabrics are more comfortable, as are clothes that are easy to put on and take off. Some women may also benefit from specialised adaptive vesture designed specifically for people with arthritis. ultimately, women with AS should know that they are not alone. Joining a support group or seeking out other women with AS can be a precious source of fellowship, advice, and goad. multitudinous online communities live for women with AS, and participating in these groups can help women feel more connected and informed about their condition. In conclusion, women with AS need to be alive of a numerous critical goods in order to manage their condition effectively. This includes understanding the impact of AS on reproductive health, bone health, emotional good, and vesture choices. also, seeking out support from other women with AS can be a precious way to stay informed and encouraged. By taking a visionary approach to their condition, women with AS can lead full and active lives while managing their symptoms

CHAPTER 17

YOUR EVERYDAY GUIDE TO LIVING WELL WITH ANKYLOSING SPONDYLITIS

Ankylosing Spondylitis(AS) is a habitual seditious complaint that affects joints in the chine. It can lead to the emulsion of the chines, performing in stiffness and pain in the reverse. The goods of the condition vary from person to person, but it can be extremely enervating and impact diurnal life. still, by making some life changes, it's possible to live well and manage the condition effectively. Then is your everyday companion to living well with Ankylosing Spondylitis .

1. Exercise regularly It may feel counterintuitive, but regular exercise can help palliate AS symptoms. It's important to engage in low- impact exercises that don't put fresh strain on joints, regularly stretching, and doing joint specific exercises. These conditioning can help increase inflexibility and range of stir, drop pain situations, and strengthen muscles. Swimming, walking or cycling are recommended as good low- impact

exercises for people with AS. Maintaining good posture and stretching during breaks at work are also recommended exercises. Exercise can also help ameliorate internal health and well- being, and reduce stress and anxiety(1).

2. Good nutrition Eating a healthy and balanced diet plays a vital part in managing AS symptoms. It's recommended to avoid foods that spark inflammation, similar as reused foods, sugar, and alcohol. rather, incorporate nutrient- thick foods like fruits, vegetables, and spare protein. Foods grandly in omega- 3, similar as fish and nuts, haveanti-inflammatory parcels and can be salutary for people with AS. It's also salutary to start the day with a good breakfast and refections rich in Vitamin D and Calcium(2).

3. Get proper sleep Fatigue is a common symptom of Ankylosing Spondylitis. Getting enough sleep at night is important in keeping energy situations over and reducing inflammation situations. contriving a sleeping routine is important; it could include relaxation ways. Sleeping on your reverse or side is recommended in order to maintain chine alignment.

4. Maintain good posture Maintaining good posture is pivotal in precluding the progression of the complaint and managing symptoms. Whether sitting or standing, it's important to avoid limping as this can put fresh strain on the chine.

5. Manage stress Stress can complicate symptoms of Ankylosing Spondylitis. Engaging in stress- reducing ways similar as contemplation or deep breathing, and taking breaks during work hours is important. Incorporating conditioning similar as gardening or reading, or pursuits like oil, writing or harkening to music can be stress- relieving as well. Managing stress helps with reducing inflammation situations and promoting better health.

6. Attend regular movables with a rheumatologist It's important to see a rheumatologist who can cover the progression of the complaint and recommend any treatment adaptations or changes. These movables should be maintained regularly and any enterprises or questions should be addressed to your healthcare provider.

7. make a support system Living with Ankylosing Spondylitis can be grueling , and having a network of support can be helpful. musketeers and family members can offer emotional support, while support groups can offer an occasion to connect with others who understand what it's like to live with the complaint. Seeking out the coffers of professional counselors is also important in managing with the habitual complaint. Living with Ankylosing Spondylitis can be a challenge, but incorporating life changes and operation strategies can extensively ameliorate quality of life. Regular exercise, good nutrition, acceptable sleep, good posture, managing stress, attending regular movables

with a rheumatologist, and erecting a support system are   each important rudiments to living well with Ankylosing Spondylitis. With these sweats, individualities can help reduce pain situations, increase inflexibility and range of stir, and manage the condition effectively.

CHAPTER 18

WHAT TO DO WHEN ANKYLOSING SPONDYLITIS GET YOU DOWN

Ankylosing Spondylitis(AS) is a habitual seditious condition that affects the chine and other joints in the body. It can beget severe pain, stiffness, and fatigue, making it challenging to carry out daily conditioning. Living with AS can be grueling , especially when the symptoms flare up. It's essential to learn how to manage with the condition and manage the symptoms effectively.   The first step to managing AS is to seek medical help. A croaker or healthcare provider can help diagnose the condition and define specifics to manage the symptoms. specifics similar as nonsteroidalanti-inflammatory medicines(NSAIDs) and corticosteroids help reduce pain and inflammation in the joints. Disease- modifying antirheumatic medicines(DMARDs) can also help decelerate down the progression of the condition.piecemeal from drug, physical remedy can also help relieve common pain and stiffness caused by AS. Physical therapists can develop an exercise program that can help ameliorate inflexibility, range of stir, and posture. Exercise can also help relieve stress, which can complicate AS symptoms. Salutary changes can also help manage AS symptoms. Eating a balanced diet with fruits, vegetables, and spare protein can help reduce inflammation, ameliorate gut health, and boost the vulnerable system. Omega- 3 adipose acids set up in fish, flaxseeds, and nuts can also help reduce inflammation in the body. Besides these medical and life changes, it's essential to maintain a positive outlook when living with AS. Living with a habitual condition can be grueling , and it can be easy to feel down and defeated. still, fastening on the effects that one can do and what makes life pleasurable can help produce a more positive outlook. It's essential to stay connected with musketeers and family and share in conditioning that bring joy and happiness.   Living with AS can also mean conforming to a new routine. It's essential to make variations to the living space and work terrain to make it easier to carry out daily conditioning. Simple variations like using a standing office, ergonomic chairpersons, and tool grips can help reduce the strain on joints.In conclusion, living with Ankylosing Spondylitis can be grueling , but there are ways to manage it effectively. Seeking medical help, maintaining a healthy life, and conforming to a new routine can help manage the symptoms and ameliorate the quality of life. With a positive outlook and a support network, it's possible to lead a happy and fulfilling life despite living with AS

CHAPTER 19

7 MYTHS ABOUT ANKYLOSING SPONDYLITIS DEBUNKED

Ankylosing Spondylitis(AS) is a rare type of arthritis that primarily affects the chine. It causes habitual inflammation of the joints, which can lead to stiffness, pain, and swelling. Unfortunately, numerous myths compass AS, which can lead to misconstructions and help people from seeking the care they need. In this essay, we will address seven of these myths and debunk them.

Myth# 1 AS is a Rare Disease,AS is frequently considered a rare complaint, but this is a myth. According to recent estimates, AS affects around0.5 of the population, making it more common than preliminarily allowed. While it's true that AS occurs less frequently than rheumatoid arthritis or osteoarthritis, it's still a significant health concern that affects thousands of people worldwide.

Myth# 2 AS is Only a Spinal Condition While AS primarily affects the chine, it can also impact other joints in the body, similar as the hips, knees, shoulders, and ankles. Some people with AS may also witness symptoms outside of the joints,similar as eye inflammation, fatigue, and bowel problems. It's important for people with AS to be apprehensive of these implicit symptoms and report them to their croaker.

Myth# 3 AS Only Affects Men AS was formerly allowed to primarily affect men, but this isn't the case. While it's true that AS is more common in men, it can also do in women. In fact, recent studies suggest that women may witness more severe symptoms and a advanced threat of disability than men with AS.

Myth# 4 AS Only Affects Aged Grown-ups, AS is frequently considered a condition that primarily affects aged grown-ups, but this isn't the case. While the symptoms of AS generally begin in early majority, the condition can do at any age, indeed in children. In fact, youngish people with AS may witness more severe symptoms and a advanced threat of disability than aged grown-ups.

Myth# 5 AS is Easy to Diagnose, AS is notoriously delicate to diagnose, and it can take several times for someone with AS to admit a proper opinion. Symptoms of AS, similar as reverse pain and stiffness, can be analogous to those of other conditions, making it challenging for croakers to identify the cause. As a result, people with AS may suffer from their symptoms for times before entering a opinion.

Myth# 6 AS Can Be Cured   Unfortunately, there's presently no cure for AS. While specifics and physical remedy can help manage symptoms, there's no way to fully exclude AS. Some people with AS may go into absolution, which means that they witness many to no symptoms for a period, but the condition can still flare up in the future.

Myth# 7 People with AS Can not Exercise Exercise is an essential part of managing AS. Regular physical exertion can help reduce pain and stiffness, ameliorate mobility, and increase overall fitness situations. While people with AS may need to modify their exercise routine to accommodate their condition, they should still be physically active whenever possible.   In conclusion, there are numerous myths girding AS that can help people from seeking the care they need. By debunking these myths and adding   mindfulness about AS, we can insure that people with this condition admit timely and effectivetreatment.However,   similar as   reverse pain and stiffness, it's essential to speak with your croaker to admit a proper   opinion and develop a treatment plan, If you're passing symptoms of AS.

CHAPTER 20

STAY HYDRATED WITH ANKYLOSING SPONDYLITIS

Ankylosing spondylitis(AS) is arthritis that affects the chine and other joints, causing pain, stiffness, and common damage. One pivotal aspect of managing this condition is staying doused . In this essay, we will bandy why hydration is important for those with AS and explore strategies to stay doused . Dehumidification is a common issue for individualities with AS. habitual inflammation can lead to fluid loss, and the specifics used to manage symptoms,similar as nonsteroidalanti-inflammatory medicines(NSAIDs), can complicate dehumidification. also, AS can affect the digestive system, leading to diarrhea and farther fluid loss. Dehumidification can worsen AS symptoms, leading to increased pain, stiffness, and fatigue. therefore, it's essential for those with AS to cover their fluid input and insure they're staying doused . Away from managing symptoms, staying doused can have other health benefits, similar as promoting healthy skin, enhancing cognitive function, and perfecting digestion. adding hydration can also prop in weight operation and drop the threat of order monuments and urinary tract infections.So how important water should someone with AS drink? The recommended diurnal input of water for the average grown-up is at least eight mugs, or 64 ounces. still, this quantum can vary depending on an existent's weight, exertion position, and climate. A person with AS may bear further water if they regularly engage in physical exertion or live in a hot and sticky terrain. also, certain specifics, similar as diuretics, can increase the need for fluids. While drinking water is essential for staying doused , there are other sources of fluids that people with AS can consume. Fruits and vegetables that have high water content, similar as watermelon, cucumber, and celery, can contribute to overall hydration situations. potables similar as herbal tea, coconut water, and low- fat milk can also give acceptable hydration. Soup and broth- grounded dishes can contribute to fluid input as well.

A way from covering fluid input, there are other strategies to insure hydration situations are maintained. One fashion is to keep a water bottle close by and drink throughout the day. Belting on fluids continuously can be more effective than staying until feeling thirsty. Adding flavor to water, similar as with bomb or lime slices, can make hydration more enticing. It may also be salutary to limit potables that can complicate dehumidification, similar as alcoholic and caffeinated drinks.In summary, staying doused is pivotal for those with AS and can prop in managing symptoms of this condition. habitual inflammation and drug use can complicate dehumidification, which can lead to worsened AS symptoms   similar as pain, stiffness, and fatigue. Drinking at least eight mugs of fluid a day and consuming fruits, vegetables, and hydrating potables can contribute to this   thing. also, covering fluid input and limiting dehumidification- converting potables can be helpful strategies. Overall, hydration is a simple yet vital aspect of managing AS symptoms and promoting overall health.

About author

DR.BEN JAPHETH is an innate member of the WHO
group . He has contributed greatly in human health and
psychological growth in the state. So he find it so helpful
to give more value to the World by putting together
some important facts about human structural framework.